Dr. Abbo's Gu
Healthy, Long Life

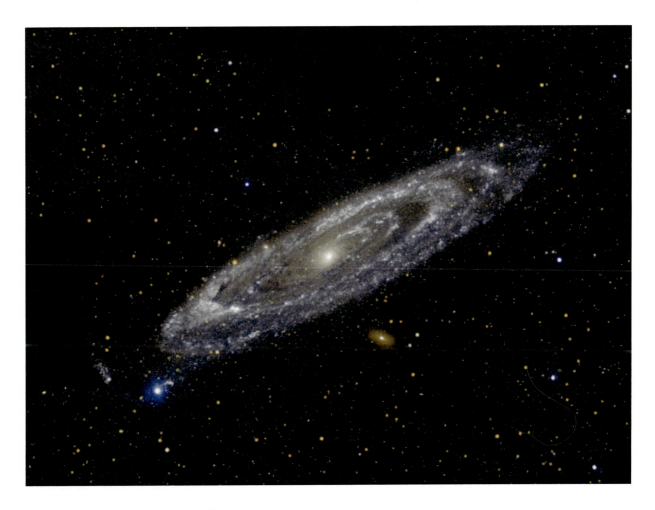

Why do we age?

How can we slow it down?

Fred E. Abbo, MD, PhD

Craig and wife,

To your good health

Fred

Copyright © Fred E. Abbo, MD. PhD 2016-2018 All rights reserved,

Andromeda Photo credit: NASA

PREFACE

Notice: This book is NOT intended to practice medicine for any individual. And it is not a Textbook of Medicine.

This book is intended for the ordinary non-medical person.

It may also be of value to doctors and medical personnel.

It focuses on general ways of helping to prevent the common diseases that occur as one grows older.

The comments and suggestions in this book are based in part on studies of large populations from various parts of the world, and may not apply for a different population group, or for any one individual.

Each person is unique ...with unique genes, metabolism, body structure, life experiences, and lifestyle.

You should check with your doctor before following any suggestion made in this book.

Some of the comments made by the author are reasonable hypotheses, based on the author's education, medical experience, logical reasoning, and judgement. However, they may not necessarily be correct.

Some health statements in this book may change with time.

Other doctors may not agree with some of the statements made in this book.

You must check with your doctor before following any suggestions made in this book, to help you decide which suggestions are right for you.

"Any logos or trademarks referenced in this book are the property of their respective owners."

The mission of this book is to help you, the reader, protect your health… as much as possible… so that you may someday benefit from the current marvelous developments in medicine, which utimately will lead to prolonging a person's healthy lifespan to an extent never before seen.

ABOUT THE AUTHOR

Fred E. Abbo, MD, PhD

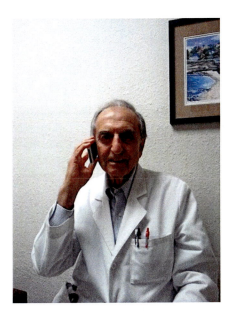

Gerontologist
 The scientific study of aging:
  Why do people grow old?
  How can we slow it down?
Practicing physician Internal Medicine
Computer programmer and designer
 President and CEO, Abbo EMR, LLC

Scientist
 Harvard, BA Chemistry, cum laude
 UC Berkeley PhD Biochemistry
 Clinical Investigator, Gerontology, V.A. Hospital, Iowa City, IA, 1963-66

Organizations:
FACP, Fellow, American College of Physicians
American Medical Association
American Aging Association
American Society for Nutrition
American Heart Association
Gerontological Society of America

ALSO BY THE AUTHOR

"**Steps to a Longer Life**" 1979

REALITY

The Universe ... infinite ... and random

with humans on an island in space ... and time ...

and the amazing creation of the awesome human brain

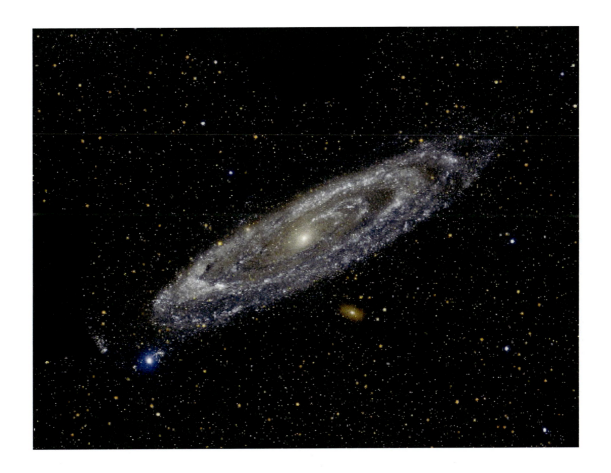

The Macro Universe ... stars and galaxies
The Micro Universe ... cells, molecules, atoms, electrons

... and humans, in the In-between Universe

The In-between Universe

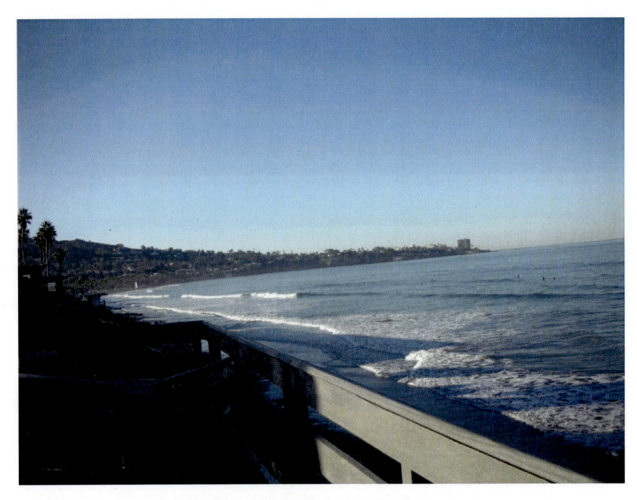

Coast off of La Jolla, California

ACKNOWLEDGMENT AND DEDICATION

***To my family, friends, and patients**, for their support and encouragement*
and
***Anybody else**, who is interested in protecting their health*

TABLE OF CONENTS

PREFACE	2
ABOUT THE AUTHOR	3
ALSO BY THE AUTHOR	4
ACKNOWLEDGMENT AND DEDICATION	7
TABLE OF CONENTS	8
THE AGE OF PREVENTIVE MEDICINE	10
HEALTH RULES OF THE BODY	11
BRAIN	14
Brain Health: Diet	14
Mediterranean diet	14
Brain Health: Physical Exercise	15
Brain Health: Mental Exercise	16
Brain Health: Executive Function	16
Brain Health: Emotions	17
Brain Health: Brain Rest	18
Brain Health: Sleep	18
Brain Risks	19
Alzheimer's Disease	20
Things that promote the risk for Alzheimer's disease:	20
Things that reduce the risk for Alzheimer's disease:	20
CANCER PREVENTION	21
DIGESTIVE SYSTEM (mouth, esophagus, stomach, intestines,…)	23
Mouth	23
Esophagus and stomach	24
Colon	25
The Intestinal Microbiome	26
Resistant Starch	26
Some sources of resistant starch:	26
EYES	28
EARS	31
HEART AND BLOOD VESSELS	32

KIDNEYS	33
LUNGS	35
NUTRITION AND DIET	36
Mediterranean Diet	36
Sugar Metabolism. Causes of Elevated Blood Sugar or A1C	36
Excess Body Fat	37
Insulin resistance	37
Vitamin C Benefits	37
Anti-inflammatory Food	38
Autophagy	38
Canola oil: The poison	40
GENITAL SYSTEM, FEMALE	42
GENITAL SYSTEM, MALE	44
MUSCLES	46
Benefits of aerobic exercise	46
SKELETAL SYSTEM: BONES AND JOINTS	47
SKIN	50
THE CAUSES OF AGING	51
Causes of excessive rate of body damage	51
Causes of insufficient repair	52
ONE - LINERS	53
LABORATORY TESTS SUGGGESTED FOR YOUR ANNUAL EXAM	61
"Track My Health" app	63

THE AGE OF PREVENTIVE MEDICINE

Medicine traditionally consisted of treating disease when it occurs.

Medicine is learning how disease develops, and how it can be prevented.

We have now entered the age of preventive medicine… how to prevent disease.

HEALTH RULES OF THE BODY

Use it or Lose it.
    Also called 'Atrophy of disuse".
    As you grow older, you "lose it" more rapidly.
    This basic rule applies to all levels of the body: from the large organs … the heart, brain, lungs, muscles … down to the cell and molecular level, involving biochemical pathways.

    On the organ level, such as the muscles, brain and joints, "Use or lose it" is generally well known. What is not generally known is that this rule applies even to small parts of the body…the muscles in and around your eyes, your vocal chords used for talking, the muscle valve that starts and stops your urination…

    If the loss does not show up until older age, it is then blamed on "aging". Examples:
- Arthritis develops when a joint is not used regularly.
- Urinary incontinence may develop if the muscle valves controlling urination become weak from disuse.
- Weakness of the voice develops in older age from infrequent talking or singing.
- Low fiber in the diet causes the muscles in the intestinal wall to weaken from decreased use, thus contributing to the development of constipation.

Evolution did not provide for a human to survive beyond the age of 25 to 30, the age before which an adult would have had children.

You can communicate with your body.
    You can listen to your body for healthful suggestions.
    You can tell your body what you want to change.

Listen to your body.

It frequently will tell you what is right or wrong, good or bad.
If you are having **pain in a muscle or joint,** your body may be telling you that you have misused that part of your body ... you have done something wrong ... and need to change it.

If you are having pain in your abdomen, your body may be telling you that you may have swallowed food or drink that is damaging to your esophagus, stomach or intestines, You may have been eating too much spices in your food, or a certain supplement or medicine.

If you are overweight... your body is telling you that you have been eating too much, or not exercising enough.

If, after eating, you feel full... your body is telling you that you have eaten too much.

If you develop cancer ... your body is telling you that you have done something wrong.
You may have done one or more of the things listed below under "CANCER PREVENTION".
So, if anything goes wrong with your health ...anything that is not a genetic problem, or not due to an accident... you can reasonably suspect that you have been doing something wrong, and, in order to remedy the problem, you need to figure out what needs to be changed.

The signals from your body are not perfect.

You can be developing a disease inside your brain, sinuses, neck, chest, esophagus, stomach, intestines, abdominal organs, joints, or other part of your body, and your body may fail to signal it in the early stages.
Examples:
 Cancer, ulcer, kidney stones, heart disease, joint disease...

In this case, the best recourse is to have thorough annual or semi-annual exams, in order to detect developing damage early.

Every person has a Chronologic age and a Biologic age.
> Chronologic age is what the calendar tells you.
> Biologic age is your real, functioning age.

Biologic age is what determines your healthful lifespan.

Most people have their own ideas of what is good and bad for their health, some of which can be wrong.
> If you have a wrong health idea, you alone will suffer the consequences of ill health.
> To help prevent this, seek expert health advice.
> Keep an open mind, and always acknowledge that some of your beliefs, and the expert's beliefs, may be wrong.

Self discipline is essential for good health.
> It is important to know what is right to do, and want to do it, but it is useless if you don't do it.
> It takes self discipline to do it… to get it done.

Too much of a good thing can be bad.
> This applies to food, medicines, herbals, supplements, and lifestyle changes… any one of which may have benefit in the short term, but cause harm in the long term.

"Positive" emotions promote good health. "Negative" emotions damage your body.
> **Positive emotions:** Humor, laughter, companionship, altruism, helping others, listening to pleasant, harmonic music…
> **Negative emotions:** Fear, anger, sorrow, loneliness, depression, pain, violence…

BRAIN

Brain Health: Diet

Follow a Mediterranean type diet.

Mediterranean diet

- Lots of vegetables, various colored vegetables, both leafy and solid.
- Fruit
- Whole grains
- Nuts, especially walnuts and almonds
- Extra virgin olive oil
- Fish, at least twice each week
- Blueberries and other berries
- Omega-3 fatty acids derived from fish. Check with your doctor regarding the proper amount for you.
- Note: Recent reports indicate that extra virgin olive oil activates a process inside brain cells (autophagy) which clears the cell trash inside brain cells and essentially restores them to a more youthful condition. These studies showed a lower incidence of Alzheimer's disease in persons given supplements of extra virgin olive oil.

Avoid:

- Large amounts of saturated fats, as in animal fat, fatty red meat
- Milk fat, cheese
- Hydrogenated fats or oils,
- Trans fats as in commercially prepared food that has been fried
- Dehydration

- As little liquid deficit as 1.5 % of your body weight, (3 glasses of water for a 150 pound person) can adversely affect your mood, memory and energy.

Comment:
> Dehydration decreases your blood volume, and thus decreases the amount of blood that flows through your body and nourishes your brain, heart and muscles. Too little salt intake may also decrease your blood volume.

- Check with your doctor as to how much liquid intake and salt is safe for you, considering your heart, kidney, liver and other organs.
- Protect your heart and blood vessels from atherosclerosis ("hardening of your arteries").
- All the measures listed here for protecting your brain also apply for protecting your heart and blood vessels, and vice versa.
- Keep your blood sugar in the optimum range.
- Alcohol, in any amount, is poison to your brain.
- Adequate intake of calcium, magnesium, vitamins C and D, and Omega-3 fatty acids from fish.
- Check the adequacy of your vitamin D intake with a blood test for it. It should be around, or slightly above, the middle of the optimum range.
- Low vitamin D blood level is associated with Alzheimer's disease and impaired mental function. Better results on brain function tests were reported associated with higher blood levels of vitamin D.

Brain Health: Physical Exercise

- Physical exercise, which requires brain activity, directly exercises the brain, and has been shown to promote the growth of new brain cells.

- All kinds of exercise are beneficial, but especially aerobic exercise, ideally 30 to 60 minutes daily.
    - Walking and jogging are natural aerobic exercises. They promote blood flow to your brain, as well as the creation of new brain cells. Lying down after exercise also helps increase blood flow to your brain.
- Swimming is excellent for promoting blood flow to your brain. But it does not provide gravitational stress on your bones, which is essential for maintaining the strength of your bones.
- Include moderate resistance exercise (weights, machines).

Brain Health: Mental Exercise

- Your brain does many things. You need to exercise all parts of your brain.
    - Use language in a variety of forms, on a variety of topics.
        - Engage your mind in local, national and world affairs.
        - Read books.
        - Listen to presentations.
        - Engage in discussions.
        - Watch good quality movies or videos.
        - Study or review school courses.
    - Listen to music, especially relaxing, melodic and inspiring music.
    - Solve meaningful and challenging problems.

Brain Health: Executive Function

- The brain executive function occurs in the front-most region of the brain, called the prefrontal cortex.
- It is involved in making plans and executing them, including long term goals … "life goals".

- It uses discipline to carry out the plan.
- Strive to make plans, and organize them into a hierarchy of goals, one goal leading to the next goal, which in turn leads to the next goal … and ultimately to a final goal.
- Brain executive function varies naturally from person to person. But it can also be developed and strengthened.
- Evolutionary significance of the forebrain: It is uniquely highly developed in humans. Brain executive function enabled humans to become the dominant animal on the planet.
- It is also involved in focus (concentrating on a topic).
- Human behavior that uses the brain's executive function reduces emotional stress, promotes happiness and good health.

Brain Health: Emotions

Minimize negative emotions
- Avoid exposing your brain to negative or unpleasant feelings and images, such as violence, evil, fear, stress or sadness.
- Negative emotions and experiences will gradually damage and eventually destroy your brain, heart, kidneys, and other tissues of your body.
- Physical exercise helps counteract emotional stress.
- Intense fear can even cause sudden cardiac death, as for example in voodoo deaths.
- A manageable amount of stress is healthy for your brain. You use your brain's problem-solving function when you manage your stresses. Your brain needs to use this function in order not to lose it.

Promote positive emotions
- Happiness … humor … happy social experiences …pleasant music … helping others who need help.

Brain Health: Brain Rest

- Rest for your brain is important.
- Strive to have a siesta every day. You don't have to actually take a nap during the siesta. Just reclining, and resting with your eyes closed is beneficial.
    - *A study in Greece showed that those persons who took a siesta regularly had a lower incidence of Alzheimer's disease.*
- Spending most of your time on one task during the day deprives those brain circuits from needed rest, just as your muscles need rest after exercise.
- Your brain has many functions. Doing a variety of things during the day allows each of those various areas of the brain that are not being used time for resting.

Brain Health: Sleep

Sleep is important, for many reasons.

- Your brain needs rest, just as your muscles do.
- Sleep helps to repair your brain, to "rejuvenate" it.
- A lack of sleep contributes to insulin resistance, which can lead to sugar abnormalities and diabetes, with all of its complications.
- A lack of sleep can contribute to depression.
- Going to sleep at irregular times has been reported to impair brain function, prematurely aging the brain "by about 7 years".
- Irregular hours of sleeping disrupts the circadian rhythm, the natural coordination of the various biochemical reactions going on in your body throughout the 24 hour day, including the various repair processes that occur during sleep.

Brain Risks

- A study reported increased risk for Alzheimer's Disease by 50% in the elderly who are taking a class of medicines called "benzodiazepines" (for example, Xanax, Ambien), for anxiety or insomnia. *(British Medical Journal, September 27, 2014).*
- Magnesium deficiency has been reported to contribute to impaired memory. In laboratory animals, magnesium deficiency produces changes consistent with Alzheimer's disease.
    - Half of Americans consume a diet deficient in magnesium.
    - Foods rich in magnesium include green leafy vegetables, whole grains and nuts.
    - Excessive alcohol ingestion tends to deplete the body stores of magnesium.
- Alcohol in any amount is a poison to the brain.
- Mercury from certain fish, such as swordfish and shark, can damage the brain.
- In a 17 year study of several thousand patients, certain commonly used medicines were found to be associated with dementia and Alzlheimer's disease. For example, *Benadryl* ® (McNeil-PPC Inc), used for sleep or allergy; chlorpheniramine, used for allergies; and oxybutynin, used for urinary problems; tolterodine, used for overactive bladder; and the tricyclic antidepressants, such as doxepin or amitriptyline. *(This study was reported in the Journal of the American Medical Association, Internal Medicine (JAMA Intern Med. Published online January 26, 2015), titled "Strongest Evidence Yet Links Anticholinergic Drugs, Dementia").*
    - **Comment**: This effect is reported for chronic (long term) use. This result is not surprising since anti-cholinergic drugs act by suppressing the formation in the brain of a chemical called "acetylcholine". This is the chemical found to be deficient in the brain cells of patients with Alzheimer's disease. And one of the medicines used to treat Alzheimer's disease acts to increase the amount of acetylcholine in the brain.

- Radiation, as from X-rays and CT scans, can damage or destroy brain cells. Caution with X-rays to the face and head.

Alzheimer's Disease

Alzheimer's disease, (and probably also Parkinson's Disease):

Things that promote the risk for Alzheimer's disease:
- Excess body fat
- Alcohol in any amount
- Magnesium deficiency
- In elderly taking certain medications for anxiety or insomnia (British medical Journal, September 27, 2014)
- Physical trauma to the head, such as blows to the head as in boxing or impact sports, excessive vibration to the head which would repeatedly bounce your brain against the inside of your skull
- Excessive blood pressure in the head, such as in exercise which keeps the head below the level of the rest of the body. This will impede the flow of blood into the brain and increase the pressure inside the skull, compressing the veins and reducing blood flow to the brain.

Things that reduce the risk for Alzheimer's disease:
- Extra virgin olive oil
- Vitamin D
- A daily siesta *(Reported in a Greek study which followed a group of individuals for 7 years, and compared those who did and did not take siestas)*
- *A* period of fasting such as after an overnight sleep, about 12 - 15 hours.
- Aerobic exercise
- Vitamin C, preferably from food, especially fruit
- Resveratrol, a chemical found in red grapes, berries, raisins and peanuts, …
- Full blood flow to any part of the body
- Autophagy. See section on Autophagy.

CANCER PREVENTION

- Follow a Mediterranean diet. See below.
- Get plenty of omega-3 fatty acids, from fish or fish oil supplements.
- Avoid being overweight.
- Don't smoke cigarettes (lung cancer). Breath clean air.
- Avoid heavy exposure to sunlight (skin cancers).
- Avoid chronic inflammation, any place in your body.
- Cancer is promoted in any part of the body where the blood flow is impaired. Massage any area of scarring.
- Avoid any intake of alcohol.
- Alcohol promotes the development of cancer of the
    - throat
    - esophagus
    - bowel
    - liver
    - breast (in women)
    - prostate
- Alcohol in the body is chemically transformed into a chemical called acetaldehyde, which is closely related to formaldehyde, a chemical used in embalming a dead person.
- Alcohol damages your DNA. Damaged DNA increases your risk for cancer.

- Avoid any charred or smoked food, especially charred meat or smoked fish.

- Optimize your vitamin D intake. Check your blood level.

- Engage in daily exercise, both aerobic and resistance exercise.

- Avoid processed meats containing nitrites (hot dogs and ham).

- **Acrylamide** is a chemical found in roasted coffee beans (**coffee**). In studies on laboratory animals, acrylamide has been found to increase the risk for cancer. California law currently designates it as a "confirmed or suspected carcinogen" (a chemical that causes cancer).

- The chemical structure of caffeine is similar to one of the chemicals naturally found in the DNA molecule (see diagrams below). It is quite likely that the caffeine molecule enters into the DNA of a person who drinks liquids containing caffeine, such as coffee, tea, cocoa and cola drinks. The incorporation of an abnormal chemical into the structure of your DNA risks the development of a disease, including cancer.

- Here are the chemical structures of caffeine and adenine, one of the four chemicals that form the structure of your DNA.
    Caffeine   Adenine

Diagrams courtesy of NIH (National Institute of Health USA)

DIGESTIVE SYSTEM (mouth, esophagus, stomach, intestines,...)

Mouth

Digestion begins in the mouth by the saliva secreted by your salivary glands. The saliva is secreted into your mouth when you chew.
If your diet is mostly liquid, your salivary glands may suffer from disuse, and you may end up with a dry mouth, susceptible to infection.

Chewing food promotes the normal secretion of saliva, which also promotes the health of your parotid glands.

Because the mouth is warm and moist, any food left in your mouth after eating or drinking promotes the growth of bacteria in the mouth.
These bacteria can cause infection of your gums and damage your teeth. They can also move down into your stomach and intestines, and cause infection there.

Rinsing your mouth with clean water before and after meals helps prevent bacterial infections in the mouth, such as gingivitis, and also lower down, in the stomach and intestines.

After-meal brushing your teeth, or rinsing between your teeth with a device that provides a stream of water between your teeth, would also help reduce the number of harmful bacteria migrating into your stomach and intestines.

Another potential health risk related to the mouth are dental X-rays. When dental X-rays are taken, a lead apron is usually placed over your chest and abdomen, to reduce your exposure to scattered X-rays. This implies that such scattered X-rays could be harmful to your health.

But, unfortunately, there is no practical way to prevent the X-rays from radiating your brain, which lies just behind and above the teeth that are being X-rayed. You should discuss with your dentist the advantages and disadvantages of dental x-rays for you, if that issue arises.

Esophagus and stomach

With increasing age. the incidence of irritation and damage to the esophagus and stomach increases.

Causes include:
- certain foods
  - black pepper
  - onions
  - lemons or limes or their juices
  - mustard
  - Other spices
- alcohol
- some medicines
- hot liquids, such as tea, coffee, cocoa, or water
- being overweight
- Lying down or sleeping within 3 hours after a meal.

Ultimately, the above chronic irritation can damage the muscular valve that separates the stomach from the esophagus, making the valve ineffective. This then allows irritating stomach contents to move upward towards your mouth and larynx and down into your lungs.

This condition is called GERD, "Gastro-Esophageal-Reflux-Disease". "Gastro" refers to the stomach. "Esophageal" refers to the swallowing tube between mouth and stomach. "Reflux" refers to the movement of some stomach contents upward into the esophagus, into the person's mouth, larynx (voice box) and lungs.

- GERD can damage your teeth, produce chronic hoarseness or chronic cough, and damage your lungs, with increased risk for pneumonia.
-
- Eating within a few hours of sleep makes a person more likely to develop "GERD".
-
- Persons with GERD may need to take medicine for the associated chronic pain.
- These medicines reduce the acid in the patients' stomach.
- Long term use of these medicines, however, can result in reduced vitamin B12 absorption, resulting in vitamin B12 deficiency and infection in the stomach and intestines.
-
- The best management for GERD is to prevent it.

Certain populations in the Pacific region who regularly drink very hot tea, have an unusuallly high incidence of cancer of the esophagus and stomach.

Colon

Common Problems: Polyps, diverticulitis (infection), infection, cancer

Causes include:

- Not enough fiber and/or liquid in the diet
- Unfriendly bacteria in the intestines, called an unfriendly "Microbiome.

The Intestinal Microbiome

Intestinal microbiome refers to the bacteria that reside in your intestines, some of which are friendly and beneficial to your health, others are harmful.
These bacteria live, grow and die in your intestines.
They release chemicals into your intestines, which may be either beneficial or harmful.
Food that you eat can affect your intestinal microbiome.

Resistant Starch

There is a special kind of starch, called "Resistant starch", which resists digestion in the small intestine and passes through into the large intestine where it is digested primarily by friendly bacteria.

When these colon bacteria digest resistant starch, they release into your colon beneficial chemicals, called short chain fatty acids.

Short chain fatty acids help prevent cancer of the colon.
Some of these short chain fatty acids are absorbed into your blood stream, and provide beneficial effects in your body.

Thus, Resistant Starch is healthful.

Some sources of resistant starch:

- Banana, raw, slightly green
- Oats, (best uncooked)
- Green peas

- Beans
- Lentils
- Corn
- Pasta
- Barley
- Potato

EYES

You have muscles in your eye structure.

To help preserve your eye function, and to stimulate the blood flow to the eye structures, you need to exercise the muscles of the eyes regularly … daily.

Eye muscle exercise promotes blood flow to the eyes, which provides nourishment and removes waste products.

Some eye-muscle exercises include:
- look far and near, left and right, up and down,
- blink your eyes, frequently (this also helps moisten your cornea).
- open your eyes widely, to exercise the eyelid opening muscles.

Avoid glare or reflection of light off of a computer screen.
Wear glare resistant glasses when working on a computer.
Keep the screen straight ahead of you, or slightly below the level of your eyes.

Avoid exposing your eyes to the sun's rays.
Sunshine, especially ultraviolet and blue light entering your eye, can damage the retina of your eye, contributing to AMD, (Adult-onset Macular Degeneration), one of the common diseases of aging, and a common cause of blindness, or loss of sharp vision.

Sun glasses can help protect your eyes against harmful ultraviolet light.

Sun glasses that absorb harmful blue light also help protect the retina of your eye. These sun glasses look yellow and give a yellow tint to the outside world.

The critical vision cells in your eye, called the "retinal pigment epithelium", need certain natural chemicals found in vegetables and fruit.

These natural chemicals include a chemical called "Lutein", considered to help prevent Adult-onset Macular Degeneration.

Another food chemical for the eye, called "Zeoxanthin", has been reported to help prevent cataract in your eye's lens.

The food rich in the above eye-beneficial chemicals include spinach, broccoli, carrots, peaches, tomatoes, citrus fruit, blueberries, cherries and raspberries.

Caution:
> **Never, ever, press on your eyeballs**, for example, when your eyes itch, or when you are tempted to squint your eyes to see better.
>
> This can tear part of your retina in your eyes … pull it right off of its normal position … producing what is called a retinal detachment, causing blindness in that part of your eye.

Positioning yourself upside down with your head lower than your feet will increase the pressure in your head, including your eyes, producing increased pressure inside your eyes.

The increased pressure on the blood vessels inside your eye reduce the blood flow to the retina lining inside your eye and eventually damages the retina in your eye.
This chronic damage to your retina, the part of your eye that receives images, can eventually produce blindness,

If you are diabetic, you should have an eye exam every year, or more often, as indicated by your eye doctor.
Diabetes increases your risk for eye disease.

If you have high blood pressure, your eyes should be checked regularly by an eye specialist.

Everybody over age 50 should have an eye exam.
After about age 60, you should have an eye exam every year, or more often as recommended by your doctor.

EARS

To reduce your risk of impairing your hearing, avoid exposing yourself to loud sound such as loud music, loud machinery, or explosions.

Skin cancers of the **pinna** of the ear (the outer structure of the ear) are common as people grow older.

You can help prevent these skin growths and cancers by rubbing the pinna daily with a face cloth, to remove the dead surface skin cells and stimulating blood flow.
Rub inside all the crevices of the pinna.

Avoid inserting a cotton tipped applicator into your ear canal in an attempt to remove accumulated wax. This only pushes the wax deeper inside the air canal, which will require removal.

HEART AND BLOOD VESSELS

- High cholesterol, high blood pressure, and abnormal sugar metabolism, are the three common causes of cardiovascular disease (heart attack, heart failure, stroke, and cardiovascular plaque in other blood vessels).

- All the suggestions made above for protecting the brain also apply for protecting the heart and blood vessels.

- Aerobic exercise, totaling about 150 minutes per week, is especially important for preventing cardiovascular disease.

- Avoid being overweight. Eliminate excess body fat, especially around your waist.

- Do not smoke.

- Maintain a normal blood pressure.

- Keep your salt intake moderate, within the recommended levels. Since the optimal level is still somewhat unsettled, check with your doctor.
  Most people get too much salt in their diet.

- But too little salt, although uncommon, can also be a problem.

- Each person is different in their salt requirements.

- Having high blood pressure or kidney disease may increase your sensitivity to salt.

- Eating a diet high in potassium, such as vegetables and fruit, helps counteract, to some extent, the harmful effect of excess salt in your diet.

KIDNEYS

Causes of kidney damage:

- Dehydration

    - If your urine is straw colored, you probably are somewhat dehydrated.

    - Dehydration reduces your blood volume. A reduced blood volume means there is a reduced supply of nourshiment and reduced removal of waste products affecting every cell in your body.

    - Dehydration may also contribute to the development of kidney stones, which can end up damaging your kidneys.

- Some medications can damage your kidneys, especially if taken for a long time:

    - Long term use of "NSAID" ("anti-inflammatory") type medicines, such as ibuprofen, celecoxib, and others.) Check with your doctor.

    - Some antibiotics. Check with your doctor.

    - Other medications. Check with your doctor.

- Obstruction to the flow of urine, as with an enlarged prostate or a kidney stone.

- Hardening of your arteries from atherosclerosis (cholesterol deposits in the arteries) or high blood pressure, which can reduce the blood flow to your kidneys.

- Heart failure can reduce the blood flow to your kidneys.

- Diabetes, not well-controlled, can damage your kidneys.

Being in the upright position too long may reduce the blood flow to the kidneys.

Diabetes can increase your risk for kidney disease.

A low vitamin D blood level increases your risk for kidney disease.

Hyperparathyroidism (overactive parathyroid glands) results when your absorption of calcium from your diet is insufficient due to either insufficient calcium intake or low vitamin D.

- When a person's intake of calcium is too low, the parathyroid glands senses it, and the parathyroid gland becomes more active ("hyper" active), in order to compensate for this calcium deficiency. An overactive parathyroid condition, however, removes calcium from the person's bones in order to maintain the normal concentration of calcium in the blood. But in the process, it weakens your bones and produces damaging calcification throughout the body … including blood vessels and kidneys. The blood tests suggested at the end of this Guide help check for this problem.

- Using the "Track My Health" app, listed at the end of this Guide below, will help you monitor all of the above tests, especially helpful in detecting an early trend in the wrong direction. You can obtain the app at this URL link: trackmyhealthapp.com

LUNGS

- There is a tendency for your lung function ... your breathing capacity ... to get weaker with age. Taking deep breaths every day, preferably through aerobic exercise, or from simple deep breathing exercise, will help slow down the weakening of your breathing muscles from disuse.

- Your heart contractions move your blood throughout your body. The blood that goes to the lower half of your body returns through your lungs. If your lungs do not function normally, through insufficient use, the blood returning to your heart from below will have a more difficult time getting through your lungs. You will then get more easily short of breath, and your entire body circulation will be impaired.

- Smoking cigarettes will eventually destroy your lungs.

- Breathing air in a room where other people are smoking cigarettes can damage your lungs.

- Carotene containing food, such as carrots, sweet potatoes, cantaloupe, and spinach, may help protect your lungs.

- Breathing polluted air, from dust or chemicals of any kind, such as asbestos, paint fumes, or smog, can damage your lungs.

- Repeated lung infections, such as bronchitis or pneumonia, can ultimately damage your lungs.

- Lung infection from certain bacteria, such as tuberculosis, or fungi, commonly will damage your lungs.

NUTRITION AND DIET

Mediterranean Diet

Lots of vegetables, various colored vegetables, both leafy and solid
Fruit
Whole grains
Nuts, especially walnuts and almonds
Extra virgin olive oil
Fish, at least twice each week
Blueberries and other berries
Omega-3 fatty acids derived from fish. Check with your doctor regarding the proper amount for you.

Sugar Metabolism. Causes of Elevated Blood Sugar or A1C

- Overweight, or weight gain over about 10 pounds
- Insufficient aerobic exercise
- Physical inactivity throughout most of the day
- Elevated blood triglycerides
- Elevated blood pressure
- Glucosamine supplement
- Sleep impaired, either in quantity or quality
- Irregular hours of sleep (called disrupting your body's circadian rhythm)
- Low vitamin B12 level
- Low blood magnesium level
- Elevated blood cortisol from emotional stress, which impairs insulin action and increases formation of sugar by the liver
- Insufficient vitamin K (best obtained from green leafy vegetables)

Excess Body Fat

Excess body fat is the result of eating too much refined carbohydrates such as sugar added to food, high fructose cane sugar, white flour such as in bread, crackers and cookies. Too little aerobic exercise adds to the problem.

Excess fat in your body enters inside the cells all over your body … your muscles, liver, kidneys, pancreas, and more … and damages those organs.

Any excess body fat that you have increases your risk for cardiovascular disease (heart attack, stroke, heart failure, blocked arteries, atrial fibrilllation), Alzheimer's disease, diabetes, high blood pressure, cancer and premature death.

Insulin resistance

The stress hormone cortisol, generated by emotional stress, impairs insulin action, called insulin resistance. This can result in higher levels of blood sugar.

Excess body fat promotes insulin resistance.

Aerobic exercise promotes insulin sensivity.

Vitamin C Benefits

Vitamin C:
- helps prevent DNA damage and cell damage through its antioxidant effect
- promotes and is essential for the synthesis of collagen throughout your body, which is essential for damage repair including ligaments, tendons, skin and blood vessels
- is essential for synthesis of brain hormones and neurotransmitters (messenger chemicals connecting one nerve with another), including serotonin, dopamine, epinephrine and norepinephrine

- may reduce the risk of cataracts and slow the progression of Macular Degeneration
- is essential for immune system function
- is essential for production of collagen in the body, which acts as a scaffold for all the cells of the body, including the skin and muscles
  - Collagen combines with elastin to provide good skin turgor (firmness).
- Vitamin C is best obtained by eating fruit.

Anti-inflammatory Food

- Green leafy vegetables
- Celery
- Broccoli
- Blueberries
- Pineapple
- Salmon and omega-3 Fish oil
- Nuts
- Extra virgin olive oil

Autophagy

Autophagy is the natural repair process present throughout your body.

Over a period of time, damage inevitably occurs inside every cell of your body.

Autophagy is an amazing natural maintenance process present in every cell of your body.

Autophagy first tries to repair any damage to the proteins and other cell structures in your cells, and recycles the useful parts of the repaired structures.

It is a natural recycling process.

If it is not able to repair the damaged structure, it labels it as "junk", and removes it from the cell. If for any reason it cannot remove the "junk" from the cell, it destroys that cell.

If the autophagy process is not able to remove this cellular "junk" or destroy that cell, disease results. Here is a list of some of those diseases:

- Alzheimer's disease
- Parkinson's disease
- heart attack
- heart failure
- stroke
- kidney disease
- muscle weakness
- muscle atrophy
- arthritis,
- intestiinal disease
- lung disease
- kidney disease
- skin disease
- and more
- In other words, it is one of the causes of what is called "aging".

Autophagy is promoted by
- a period of fasting such as after a night's sleep, about 12 to 15 hours without food
- aerobic exercise
- extra virgin olive oil
- vitamin C
- resveratrol, a chemical found in red grapes, raisins, berries and peanuts
- full blood flow to any part of the body

When the rate of damage occurring in any part of the body is greater than the rate of repair, the accumulated damage is commonly attributed to "Aging".

Canola oil: The poison

Canola oil is a highly processed vegetable oil from the rapeseed plant, which contains trans fats and a poison called **erucic acid**.

However, canola oil has had a reputation for being harmless, and even having health benefits. It is currently very popular and is in wide use.

The content of erucic acid is currently considered to be insignificant.

For example, in an article published by the Mayo Clinic in the year 2009 on the question of canola oil containing a toxin (poison), the following conclusion was expressed:

"… **Canola oil, however, contains very low levels of erucic acid.**"
also
"… Canola is generally recognized as safe by the Food and Drug Administration."

Reference: "Zeratsky, Katherine (2009). "Canola Oil: Does it Contain Toxins?". Mayo Clinic."

Comment: Though there may be ("only") "low levels of erucic acid" in canola oil, what is overlooked is how widespread canola oil is used in our food.
For example, it is used in popular liquid nutritional drinks; as a coating for fish; in salad dressings, bread, soups, and more.

Also, a "**small amount**", means a "**small concentration**".

But in a large volume, for example one cup of a liquid dietary supplement containing canola, when taken one or more times daily, a "small amount" becomes a **large amount,**

Erucic acid prevents the cells in your body from burning fat for energy.

Harmful effects from canola oil:

- When you exercise, you will feel weak, and unsteady, for no apparent reason.
- If you are on a weight reducing diet, trying to lose excess body fat, it will be very difficult for you to succeed.
- It promotes the formation of scar tissue in your heart, weakening your heart's pumping action. This, in turn, reduces the flow of blood all over your body, which slowly damages every part of your body.
- Frail, elderly persons commonly drink liquid nutritional supplements for their nourishment. Many of these popular liquid nutritional supplements contain canola oil. The frail, elderly person's gradual worsening condition will be blamed on "aging", when in fact it is the canola oil that is causing their worsening condition.

Remebber, canola is widely used.
Check the INGREDIENTS label in the food in your home and food market, to see which foods contain canola.

Any amount of a poison in your diet is harmful.

Canola oil should be excluded from your diet.

GENITAL SYSTEM, FEMALE

Infection is largely related to a person's personal hygiene and sexual contact. Use protection when indicated. Consult with your Gynecologist.

Cancer of breast and pelvic organs are a complex, individual issue, best managed by your Gynecologist.

Urinary Incontinence can be managed, in many women, with Kegel exercises.

There are many different forms of Kegel exercises. One form is the following regimen:

Kegel Exercises

While sitting on a toilet seat or chair, standing, or in your car waiting for the red light:
- Contract your bladder and rectal muscles tightly and hold for one second. Rest for one or two seconds.
- Repeat for a total of 10 - 20 repetitions.
- Do not take much less or much more time than one second for each contraction, for maintaining optimum blood flow to the involved muscles.
- Repeat throughout the day.

Note: In order to **prevent urinary incontinence** rather than waiting until the problem develops, Kegel exerises ideally should be started when a person reaches full adulthood, about age 30, and continued for life.

Hormonal issues are still a controversial, complex, **individual** issue, best managed by your Gynecologist.

However, over the many years that I have practiced medicine, I have noticed that those post-menopausal women who were taking female hormone supplements had a definite younger appearance than those not on hormone supplements.
Check with your own doctor on this issue as it applies to you personally.

Genetic issues are a complex, **individual** issue, best managed by your Gynecologist.

Regular annual or semi-annual exams by your Gynecologist or primary doctor are essential.

GENITAL SYSTEM, MALE

Infection is largely related to a person's personal hygiene and sexual contact. Use protection when indicated.

Prostate enlargement
Avoid sexual arousal without completion.
Periodic release of normal, prostatic secretions.

Cancer of the prostate
Prevention:
- Low-fat diet, especially avoiding animal fat
- Lots of fruits and vegetables in the diet
- Fish in diet
- Reduce dairy products
- Supplement of Omega-3 fatty acids from fish
- Avoid being overweight
- Kegel exercises, to promote increased blood flow to the muscles surrounding the prostate. See below.
- Caution with bicycle riding. If the seat is small, that will put pressure on the region of the prostate, which reduces the flow of blood to the prostate.
  - Diminished blood flow to any part of the body increases the risk for development of cancer to that part of the body.
- Release of normally accumulated prostate secretions through periodic sexual activity. Note: The optimum frequency of sexual activity with release of prostatic secretions has not been scientifically determined.
- Annual PSA test and digital rectal exam ("DRG") beginning about age 45.

Urinary Incontinence
For prevention, perform Kegel exercises regularly, beginning about age 30.

Kegel Exercises

- While sitting on a toilet seat or chair, standing, or in your car waiting for the red light:
    - Contract your bladder and rectal muscles tightly and hold for one second. Rest for one or two seconds.
    - Repeat for a total of 10 - 20 repetitions.
    - Do not take much less or much more time than one second for each contraction, for maintaining optimum blood flow to the involved muscles.
    - Repeat throughout the day.

    Recommended: regular exams by your Urologist or primary care doctor beginning at age 50.

MUSCLES

To improve muscle strength, all you need is to do enough repetitions to make yourself tired, irrespective of the amount of resistance with each repetition.

My suggestion is to use the amount of dumbbell weight that allows you to do something like 20 to 30 repetitions at one time without straining.

Benefits of aerobic exercise

- Reduces the risk for cardiovascular disease (heart attack, heart failure, stroke, hardening of the arteries)
- Reduces blood pressure
- Reduces risk for diabetes
- Reduces risk for fractures
- Improves immune system, to fight infections and reduces the risk of developing cancer
- Promotes the devlopment of new brain cells
- Increases the level of the "feel good" brain chemicals, called "endorphins"
- Reduces risk for depression and anxiety
- Enhances the quality of sleep, including important deep sleep
- Enhances blood flow to the brain
- Enhances mental acuity
- Enhances sex drive
- Helps maintain normal weight
- Prolongs healthy lifespan

SKELETAL SYSTEM: BONES AND JOINTS

Exercise

Physical exercise should include aerobic, resistance, balance, and stretching exercises.

Regular aerobic exercise is essential for maintaining the health of your bones and joints. The exercise should provide gravitational stress on your bones, in which your muscles and joints are working against gravity,

Walking and jogging are probably the most natural forms of exercise.

Ideally, the exercise program should involve all the muscles and joints of your body.

Strive for aerobic exercise 150 minutes per week and resistance exercise two or three times a week.

Resistance exercises should be performed slowly…for each rep, about one second for the contraction phase, and one second for the muscle relaxation phase. Number of reps: 20 - 30

Bone Health

The level of vitamin D in your blood should be measured regularly and be kept in the optimal range. This is the only way to be sure that you are getting enough vitamin D to keep your bones strong.

You cannot rely on exposure of your skin to sunlight to provide you with your optimum amount of vitamin D.
The effectiveness of sunlight on your skin in promoting the synthesis of vitamin D varies from person to person, and diminishes with age.

Your calcium intake is important for maintaining your bones and joints. For middle-aged and older adults, your total daily intake should be approximately 1000 - 1200 milligrams.

If you need to take supplements of calcium in order to maintain the required intake, keep in mind that you cannot absorb more than 500 mg of calcium at any one feeding.

Do not take magnesium at the same time that you take calcium, because these two elements compete with each other for absorption through your intestines. If you are taking both supplements, they should be taken at separate times.

Joint health:

In a joint, the space between the two bones contains a cartilage that acts as a cushion.
Caution: Cartilage in joints do not have blood vessels in them. Cartilage requires intermittent compression and relaxation, like squeezing and relaxing a sponge, in order to move essential nutrients into, and waste products out of, the cartilage.

If you stand still for more than a few minutes, you are compressing the cartilage in your leg joints without this important pumping action, and, in time, your joints will deteriorate. You may end up requiring joint replacement.

Being overweight hastens the damage.

Some occupations, such as salespersons, grocery check out persons, barbers and hairdressers, thus risk ultimately damaging their joints.

Joints that are not regularly put through their full possible range of motion, will ultimately deteriorate and result in what is called "arthritis".
> Examples include the joints in the neck, shoulders, elbows, wrists, fingers, ankles and toes.

Prevention consists of putting these joints through their full range of motion regularly, on a daily basis.

SKIN

Application of ointments to the skin allows absorption of the chemicals that are dissolved in the ointment to be absorbed through the skin into the body, to spread and cause damage throughout the body.

Massaging your skin regularly, for example with your towel after a shower, has beneficial effects. It helps remove the dead surface skin cells, which, if not removed, will cause deterioration of the skin, growths, and possibly cancer.

The skin massage also promotes blood flow to the area between the skin and underlying muscle, whitch containds supportive fibrous tissue.

If not regularly massaged, this normal fibrous tissue will deteriorate and produce wrinkles in your skin.

Vitamin C is involved in synthesising new fibrous tissue beneath the skin. Vitamin C is best obtained by eating fruit.

THE CAUSES OF AGING

The body has powerful, complex, built-in mechanisms for repair of body damage, including autophagy.
However, **the rate of repair** may not keep up with t**he rate of damage**.

The rate of repair may be different in each organ of the body.
   For example, in one person, the rate of damage may be faster in the lungs than in any other organ of the body. In another person, it may be the heart, or the blood vessels, or the kidney, or any other organ or tissue.

"Aging" is the accumulation of body damage faster than it is repaired.

Causes of excessive rate of body damage

- Excess body fat
    - Producing diabetes, high blood pressure, heart disease, stroke, insulin resistance, low HDL cholesterol
- Accidents
- Too much disuse atrophy ("Use it or lose it")
- Misuse of parts of the body
    - Sports causing trauma to the head, joints, muscles or tendons
- Risky exposure to infectious bacteria, viruses or parasites
- Deeply emotionally traumatic experiences as a child, that are not corrected over time, causing damage to the brain
- Chronic negative emotions and experiences
    - Anger, fear, solitude, stress, violence, …
- Low amount of positive emotions and experiences
    - Examples: Love, empathy, humor, companionship, music …
- Insufficient rest or relaxation
- Indoctrination of enduring, erroneous, health-damaging ideas as a child

- Deficiency of certain vitamins, for example vitamins C, D, K, folic acid, vitamins B6, and B12, and possibly others
- Inactivity, both physical and mental
- Acquiring wrong ideas about how to keep healthy. (Medical misinformation, which is common)
- Exposure to a harmful environment … either polluted air, including cigarette smoke and asbestos, radiation, excessive heat or cold, sound, light
- Ultraviolet rays, body vibrations, blunt trauma such as with boxing or impact sports

Causes of insufficient repair

- Insufficient stimulation of the body's autophagy repair process
- Genetic (DNA) damage, congenital or acquired, not recognized or treated as a genetic problem
    - Low vitamin B12, B6 or Folic Acid
    - Too much caffeine in the diet
    - X-rays and other radiation
- Impaired blood flow, reducing the delivery of normal body repair chemicals or particles
    - Insufficient aerobic exercise
- Poor diet
- Anemia
- Low oxygen in the blood from various causes
- High exposure to polluted air
- Low number of platelets (platelets in your blood have a repair function).

ONE - LINERS

One-liners are brief bits of significant medical information, derived from a variety of sources, or a new medical hypothesis from the author, Dr. Fred Abbo.

"We are what we do repeatedly" — *Aristotle, about 2300 years ago*

Arthritis pain tends to make you less active. The inactivity only makes the joint stiffer and more painful. It also contributes to balance problems. It's a vicious cycle that should be broken.

Diminished brain tissue has been found to be associated with prediabetes, in which your fasting blood sugar is slightly high.
This indicates that the separation between prediabetes and diabetes is not a sharp line, but a gradual change, and diabetic damage occurs before you have the diagnosis of diabetes.

Physical activity improves non-alcoholic fatty liver disease.

Beans, peas, lentils, and other legumes are rich in fiber, folic acid, potassium and magnesium. They also tend to lower "bad" LDL cholesterol, help lower blood pressure because of their potassium and magnesium content, and promote regularity in bowel function. They have high fiber content compared to other vegetables.

Brain cells use primarily glucose as their source of energy. A diet extremely low in carbohydrates may be harmful to the brain.

Brain cells use up a lot of energy but are not able to store energy.

Brain cells are very sensitive to slightly decreased circulation in their small blood vessels.

Aerobic exercise 150 minutes per week and resistance exercise two or more times a week will help rejuvenate your brain.

From the evolutionary and biological point of view, the chimpanzee is the closest animal to humans,
- Chimpanzees usually die of the consequences of **myocardial fibrosis (scarring of the heart)**, not coronary artery disease.
- This may be because they are in captivity and consequently under continuous emotional stress.
- It is probably the chronic stress of captivity that is killing chimpanzees prematurely before they develop coronary artery disease.
- This probably is the result of the harmful effect of chronic stress.

Primitive man reportedly ate mostly fruit.

Our DNA evolved while being exposed to natural foods, not manufactured food.

Alcohol, as used by modern man, is not a natural food.

Some things can be beneficial over a short period of time, but harmful over a longer period of time .
For example, some herbals can have a beneficial effect in the short-term, and a harmful effect over the long term.

A high level of sugar intake promotes the attachment of sugar molecules to proteins all over your body, damaging the proteins, and impairing their function.

To some extent, your body can repair these damaged proteins, but prolonged high blood sugar will result in residual damage.

Eating foods slowly, rather than rapidly, reduces the rise in blood sugar after a meal.

Not all natural foods are healthy.

Some natural foods are poisons.

The hippocampus is the area of the brain involved in memory and consciousness.
- It **decreases** in size with age.
- A study of sedentary men and women age 50 to 80 who started walking 40 minutes three days a week for six months, showed that the volume or size of their hippocampus **increased**.

High dietary fiber intake is associated with better kidney function and reduced risk for intestinal cancer.

Whole grain in the diet three times a day is reported to be associated with prolonged healthy longevity, with reduced incidence of common chronic age related diseases.

Resistant starch should be a daily part of your diet.

Drinking water with each meal and whole grain fiber promotes healthy intestinal function and a healthy microbiome.

Warm-up time varies between individuals. After prolonged inactivity of many months, the warm up time required may be prolonged.

The pumping action for circulating the blood is mediated not only by the heart, but also by the lungs, particularly with deep abdominal breathing, and contractions of the muscles of the leg, especially the calf muscles.

A chronic diastolic blood pressure below 60 is associated with damage to the heart.

A chronic heart rate over approximately 80 beats per minute will gradually damage the heart.
- The reason for this is that a fast heart beat does not allow enough time for the blood to enter your heart muscle. Your heart muscle then gradually is starved, and the heart's waste products don't have enough time to be removed.

Prebiotics feed the favorable probiotic bacteria that are present in your intestines.
- Prebiotics include bananas, oatmeal, red wine, honey, maple syrup, asparagus and peas.

In general, your longevity is inversely proportional to the amount of sitting that you do.

Calorie restriction promotes longevity by reducing the density of free radicals and free electrons in the cell.
The extent of the added longevity, however, is limited to about 25%.

The average American gets about 300 millirems of radiation a year from background sources such as the sun and cosmic radiation.
A chest x-ray provides a few millirems.
A cross country airplane ride provides about 5 millirems.

Epidemiologic evidence reportedly supports a causal association of alcohol consumption and cancers of the oropharynx, larynx, esophagus, liver, colon, rectum, and female breast.

Tau protein inside brain nerve cells (neurons) are essential for the normal working of those brain cells.
- The autophagy process removes damaged tau proteins…cell "trash".
- Damaged tau protein in brain nerve cells is highly correlated with development of Alzheimer's disease.
- Impaired autophagy in the brain contributes to the development of Alzheimer's and Parkinson's disease.
- Impaired brain function is closely correlated with the degree of tau damage.

Exercise, especially after a night's sleep, and extra Virgin olive oil, both promote autophagy.

Vitamin C is essential for the health of collagen throughout the body.
- But too much vitamin C, from supplements, can be harmful.
- A large American study of 10,000 patients suggested that the optimum serum vitamin C concentration was 53 to 70 $\mu mol/liter$ with respect to the occurrence of back pain or neck pain in the past three months.

For optimum brain function, the brain needs a constant supply of nutrients including mostly carbohydrates but also some protein and healthy fats.
It also requires rest periods throughout the day, which means varying the kind of activity that it engages in.

Average sodium intake is 3 to 6 grams per day.

- Less than 3 g per day is reportedly associated with increased risk of cardiovascular events and death regardless of high blood pressure or normal.
- Sodium intake above 6 g per day reportedly increases risk only in patients with high blood pressure, heart failure, or a kidney disease.

Some scientists believe shortening of DNA telomeres (on the ends of chromosomes) leads to aging and earlier death.
- Androgens, such as testosterone, may help prevent shortening of DNA telomeres, and may even promote prolongation of them.

Sustained aerobic exercise, but not resistance exercise or high intensity anaerobic exercise, promoted new brain cells (hippocampal neurogenesis) in laboratory rats.

Metformin, a medicine commonly prescribed for diabetes, reduces the blood level of vitamin B12.
- If you are taking Metformin, have your blood level of vitamin B12 checked regularly.
- However, Metformin has some important beneficial effects, including possible prevention of cancer.

Omega-3 fatty acids are found in:
- high amount in walnuts but not in almonds.
- walnut oils
- spinach
- fish

Plant Omega-3 fatty acids reportedly are anti-inflammatory.
The fish omega-3 fatty acids are found especially in salmon, tuna, herring, lake trout, sardines, and halibut.

A randomized controlled trial showed that 2.5 g daily of omega-3 fatty acids resulted in lower measures of inflammation and oxidative stress in humans as well as longer DNA telomeres.

Studies suggest that dark chocolate improves blood vessel flow and may improve blood sugar levels and insulin sensitivity.
However, dark chocolate contains caffeine, which can stimulate heart rhythm abnormalities, and possibly damage your DNA.

Optimum blood levels of vitamin D, above 40, are associated with approximately 65% reduction in the incidence of various cancers.

A study showed that elderly persons who were able to stand on 1 foot unassisted for 15 seconds had increased longevity and 85% diminished risk for falls.

Foods that can reduce stress:
- Oatmeal, promotes production of serotonin.
- All carbohydrates promote production of serotonin, a brain chemical.
  - Serotonin promotes memory, learning, sleep, sex drive, good mood,
  - Simple carbs do it also, but be careful for their sugar effect.
- Vitamin C reduces the level of stress hormones such as adrenaline and cortisol.
- Keep your magnesium level high.
  - Spinach and other leafy, green vegetables are high in magnesium.
- Omega-3 fatty acids reduce stress hormone levels.
- Nuts such as walnuts, almonds, and pistachios, one handful daily, reduce inflammation and risk for diabetes and protect against stress.
- Calcium reduces stress.

Vitamin K is essential for the incorporation of calcium into bone.
- Low levels of vitamin K weaken bones and promote calcification of arteries and other soft tissues.
- Vitamin K is synthesized by plants and is found in highest amounts in green leafy vegetables.

Fructose can cause diarrhea, especially in children.
- Apple and pear juice have a high concentration of free fructose.
- Maple syrup is low in fructose.

Balance training exercise helps reduce the risk of injurious falls in the elderly.
It may take one or two years to get the benefit.

Vitamin K depletion increases risk for vitamin D toxicity, and vice versa.

Vitamin D is important in promoting healthy bones, reducing cancer, fighting infections, and enhancing the immune system.

Chronic stress promotes the release of adrenaline, which has harmful effects on the cardiovascular system and promotes cancer, including ovarian cancer.

LABORATORY TESTS SUGGGESTED FOR YOUR ANNUAL EXAM

To track your progress in your effort to improve your health, consider getting the valuable app, "Track My Health". See below for details.

<u>Comprehensive Metabolic Panel</u>
Includes, among other tests, fasting blood sugar (reflets insulin sensitivity and risk for diabetes), protein, albumen (for protein metabolism), liver tests SGPT and SGOT, calcium, creatinine for kidney function,, sodium and potassium,

<u>NMR Lipoprofile (Lipid Profile)</u>
measures not only the usual choiesterol, HDL, Triglycerides and LDL, but also the important small dense LDL

<u>CBC with differential, with Platelets</u>
measures for infection, anemia, leukemia, and platelets for normal clotting and normal repair

<u>hs cardiac CRP</u>
a very sensitive test for inflammation any place in your body, including the lining of your arteries

<u>Hemoglobin A1C</u>
measures the sugar level in your blood over the preceding 2 months, and risk for diabetes

<u>Magnesium</u>
important for bone structure and energy enzymes throughout the body, including sugar metabolism

<u>ProBNP (sometimes called "NT- ProBNP ")   (only if over age 49)</u>
detects early changes in your heart muscle leading to heart failure, and the severity of heart failure

<u>PSA (only for males over age 49)</u>
detects prostate enlargement, infection or cancer

<u>Cortisol</u>
reflects *the level of your emotional stress*

<u>Ferritin</u>
detects early iron deficiency or iron overload

<u>Testosterone, Total and Free</u>
promotes buildup of body tissue and sense of energy

TSH and Free Thyroxine T4
reflects level of body metabolism

Vitamin D, 25-Hydroxy
important for absorbing calcium from your diet, maintaining your bone structure, and supporting your immune function

Vitamin B12
important for maintaining the normal functioning of the nerves in your brain as well as throughout your body. Also important for producing energy in every cell of your body, and a general sense of energy.

Homocysteine
A measure of risk for damaging your DNA due to deficiency of folic acid, vitamin B6, or vitamin B 12

PTHi (Parathyroid hormone intact)
detects insufficient calcium absorption, which causes overactivity of the parathyroid gland, called "hyperparathyroiism". Hyperparathyroiism removes calcium from your bones and moves the calcium into your blood stream, thus weakening your bones. This hyperparathyroidism promotes calcification in your arteries, kidneys and other body tissues.

Uric acid, (serum)
detects impaired liver metabolism and risk for gout

Urinalysis (Culture if positive)
detects infection, bleeding or cancer in the urinary tract

Occult blood, Fecal, IA (ImmunoAssay)
detects occult (unnoticeable) bleeding not only from your colon, but also from your esophagus, stomach and small intestine. A colonoscopy only checks your colon

Urine microalbumin/creatinine ratio
detects kidney damage and damage to the lining of your arteries, including the capillaries throughout your entire body

Osteocalcin
measures whether your bones are building normally. If they are not, you are at risk for developing osteoporosis, a weakening of your bones, with increased risk for bone fractures.

===

Notice

The **second edition** of this Guide will be published in January 2019, incorporating any significant new developments in preventive medicine.

Look for it in **amazon.com**, or your own favorite bookstore.

===

Now that you are on your way to better health, you need a way of tracking your health.
We have just the solution for that… our app:

"Track My Health" app

Available on the Apple app store. Use this link: trackmyhealthapp.com
With this app, you can see how your medicines, supplements and lifestyle changes are affecting your health.

- You enter your lab test results, medications, supplements and lifestyle changes.
- The lab test results automatically display on a graph.
  You can track their trend on the graphs.
- There is no limit to the length of the graphs of any particular lab test.
- You can see the effect of your medications, supplements and lifestyle changes at any point in time on the graph, by simply tapping on that data point.
  - A box will appear, telling you what your medicines, lifestyle changes and herbals were at that point in time.
  - This valuable function is unique, protected by a patent pending.

To see a 5-minute tutorial video of the TMH (Track My Health) app,

1. go to this URL link: trackmyhealthapp.com
2. Tap on "Watch Video"
3. When the video starts, tap in the right lower corner to enlarge the video to full screen.
4. To terminate, tap "Esc" key.
5. It's best to view the video on a larger screen, such as an iPad, desktop or lap top computer.

To purchase the app:
1. go to this URL link: trackmyhealthapp.com
2. Tap on "Available on the app store".

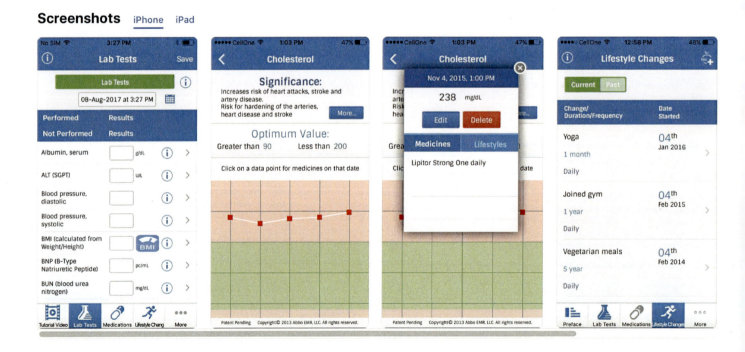

Made in the USA
San Bernardino, CA
21 June 2018